Helicobacter Pylori Antidote Handbook Made Easy:

Full Guide on H. Pylori Cure; Causes; Symptoms, Diagnosis & Treatments (Plus Natural Solutions); Includes Remedies for H. Pylori-Related Peptic Ulcer & So on

By

Dr. Jordan W. Galway

Copyright@2020

TABLE OF CONTENTS

CHAPTER ONE

INTRODUCTION

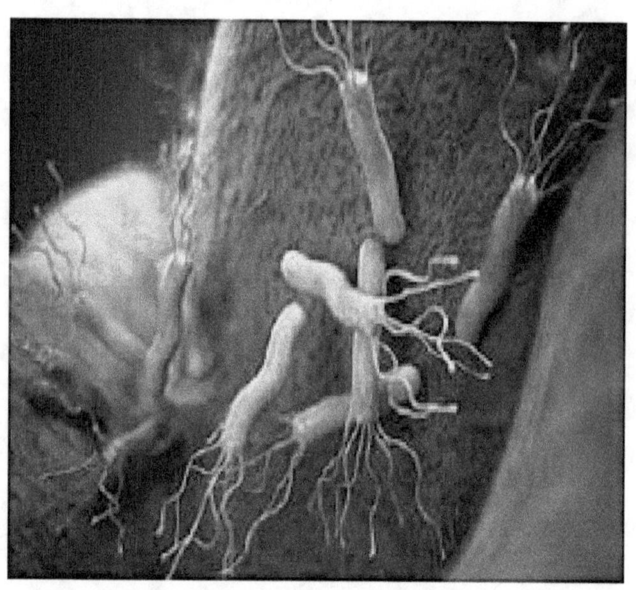

The essentials

Helicobacter pylori (H. pylori) are microscopic organisms that taint the covering of your stomach. As per 1998 information from the Centres for Disease Control and Prevention (CDC), these microorganisms are liable for up to 80 percent of gastric ulcers and 90 percent of duodenal ulcers. These might lead to certain stomach challenges, such as:

-consuming torment in the midsection

-swelling

-queasiness

-loss of craving

-successive burping

-unexplained weight reduction

The utilization of regular medicines like anti-microbial can be hard for certain individuals. It's conceivable to encounter negative symptoms, for example, queasiness, loose bowels, loss of hunger. A couple of individuals are impenetrable against microbial, which can ensnare standard approaches to manage treatment. Accordingly, enthusiasm for normal medicines is developing.

Again, H. pylori is a typical kind of microscopic organisms that develops in the stomach related plot and tends to assault the stomach lining. It taints the stomachs of about 60 percent of the world's grown-up populace. H. pylori contaminations are generally innocuous, yet they're answerable for most of ulcers in the stomach and small digestive tract.

The **H** in the name represents Helicobacter. **Helico** means winding, which reveal that the microscopic organisms are snaky formed.

H. pylori regularly taint your stomach during youth. While defilements with this strain of organisms customarily don't cause symptoms, they can incite sicknesses in specific people, including peptic ulcers, and a provocative condition inside your stomach known as gastritis.

H. pylori are accustomed to stay in very nasty, acidic state of the very stomach. These microbes can change nature around them and lessen its acridity so they can endure. The winding state of H. pylori permits them to infiltrate your stomach lining, where they're secured by bodily fluid and your body's insusceptible cells can't contact them. The microorganisms can meddle with your safe reaction and guarantee that they're not demolished. This can prompt stomach issues.

The next chapters tell you all you need to know about Helicobacter Pylori Cure; including using natural means and medications, and so on.

CHAPTER TWO

PERSONS WHO ARE AT RISKS OF THE DISEASE, PHOTOTHERAPY, AND CUSTOMARY MEDICINES FOR H. PYLORI DISEASE

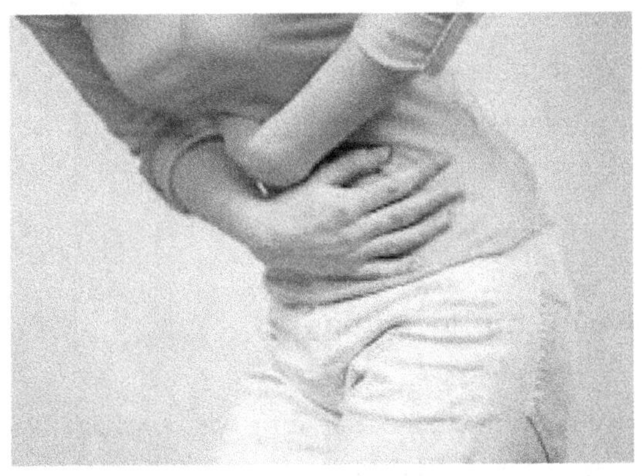

Who is in danger for H. pylori disease?

Youngsters are bound to build up a H. pylori contamination. Their danger is higher generally because of absence of legitimate cleanliness.

The danger for disease incompletely relies upon your condition and everyday environments. Your danger is higher in the event that you:

Live in a nation that is developing

Share lodging with other people who are contaminated with H. pylori

Live in stuffed lodging

Have no admittance to boiling water, which can assist with keeping territories spotless and liberated from microbes are of non-Hispanic Black or Mexican American are tolerable.

It's presently perceived that peptic ulcers are brought about by this kind of microbes, instead of stress or eating nourishments high in corrosive. And long haul utilization of nonsteroidal enemy of inflammatories (NSAIDs) likewise expands your danger of getting a peptic ulcer.

Modern research shows that H. pylori are powerless against light. Phototherapy utilizes bright light to help take out H. pylori in the stomach. Specialists accept phototherapy utilized inside the stomach is protected. It might be most valuable when anti-microbials are impossible.

Customary medicines for H. pylori disease

Specialists regularly recommend a mix of two anti-toxins and a corrosive diminishing medication to treat H. pylori. This is known as triple treatment.

In case you're impervious to the anti-infection agents, your PCPs may add another prescription to your treatment plan. The goal is to discard 90 percent or a more noteworthy measure of the H. pylori microorganisms present.

Treatment as a rule keeps going close to about fourteen days. Utilizing two anti-toxins rather than one may decrease your danger of anti-toxin opposition. Anti-microbial used to treat H. pylori include:

-amoxicillin

-antibiotic medication

-metronidazole

-clarithromycin

Corrosive diminishing prescriptions help your stomach coating to mend. A portion of these are:

-proton siphon inhibitors, for instance, lansoprazole, and omeprazole (Prilosec) - (Prevacid), which discontinue corrosive creation in the human stomach

-histamine blockers, for instance, cimetidine (Tagamet), which square corrosive setting off histamine

-bismuth subsalicylate (Pepto-Bismol), which covers and secures the coating of your stomach

More Detailed Explanations on the Drugs

You will typically need to take a blend of two distinct anti-toxins, along with another medication that decreases your stomach corrosive. Bringing down stomach corrosive enables the anti-toxins to work all the more successfully. This treatment is now and again alluded to astriple treatment.

A portion of the medications that are utilized in a triple treatment include:

-clarithromycin

-proton-siphon inhibitors; PPI, for instance, esomeprazole (Nexium), lansoprazole (Prevacid), rabeprazole (AcipHex), or even pantoprazole (Protonix).

-metronidazole (for 7 to 14 days)

-amoxicillin (for 7 to 14 days)

Therapy may differ contingent upon your past clinical history and in the event that you have hypersensitivities to any of these prescriptions.

After treatment, you will have a subsequent test for H. pylori. Much of the time, just one round of anti-infection agents is expected to clear the disease; however you may need to take more, utilizing various medications.

CHAPTER THREE

NATURAL CURES FOR HELICOBACTER PYLORI DISEASE

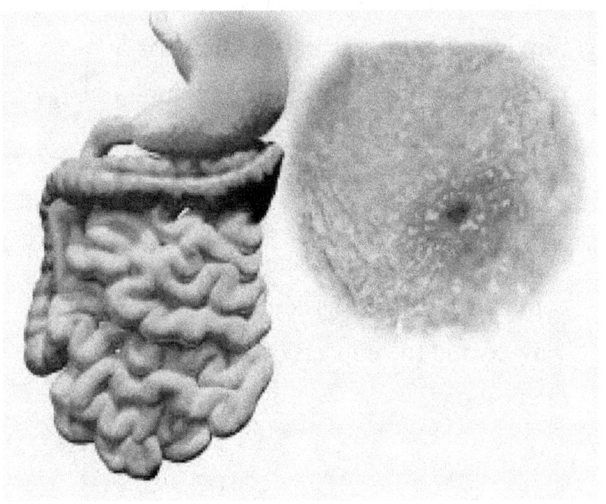

Numerous in vivo and in vitro investigations on normal H. pylori medicines have been finished. Most medicines diminished the quantity of microorganisms in the stomach however neglected to for all time kill them.

Make certain to chat with your primary care physician before starting a characteristic treatment routine. You shouldn't trade your suggest treatment for H. pylori with characteristic cures.

With your PCP's endorsement, you can utilize common medicines as adjuvant treatment. This may expand the impacts of ordinary medications.

Probiotics

Probiotics help keep up the harmony among great and terrible gut microbes. Modern studies reveal that taking probiotics previously or after standard H. pylori treatment may improve annihilation rates. Anti-microbials slaughter both great and terrible microorganisms in your stomach. Probiotics help renew great microscopic organisms. They may likewise decrease your danger of creating yeast abundance. Specialists discovered proof to propose that the microorganism Lactobacillus acidophilus conveys the best outcomes.

Green tea

Recent studies on mice indicated that green tea may help slaughter and moderate the development of Helicobacter microorganisms. The examination found that expending green tea before a disease forestalls stomach aggravation. Expending the tea during a contamination decreased the seriousness of gastritis. Locate an extraordinary choice of green tea here.

Honey

Honey has demonstrated antibacterial capacities against H. pylori. Extra examination bolsters this end. No examination to date has indicated that nectar can annihilate the microbes all alone. Analysts propose that utilizing nectar with standard medicines may abbreviate treatment time. Crude nectar as well as manuka nectar are having mainly antibacterial results.

Olive oil

Olive oil may likewise treat H. pylori microbes. A recent report showed that olive oil has solid antibacterial abilities against eight H. pylori strains. Three of those strains are anti-microbial safe. Olive oil additionally stays stable in gastric corrosive.

Licorice root

Licorice root is a typical common solution for stomach ulcers. It might likewise battle H. pylori. As indicated by a recent report, licorice root doesn't legitimately slaughter the microscopic organisms; however it can help keep it from adhering to cell dividers. There are assortments of choices accessible for buy on the web.

Broccoli sprouts

A compound in broccoli sprouts called sulphoraphane might be powerful against H. pylori. Examination on mice and people proposes that it diminishes gastric irritation. It furthermore lessens microscopic organisms' migration plus its possessions. A recent study on individuals with both sort 2 diabetes and H. pylori demonstrated that broccoli sprout powder battles the microbes. It likewise improved cardiovascular danger factors.

CHAPTER FOUR

STANDPOINT OF H. PYLORI, WHAT CAN BE DONE BY YOU AND HOW TO PREVENT FUTURE SCENARIOS OR CONTAMINATION

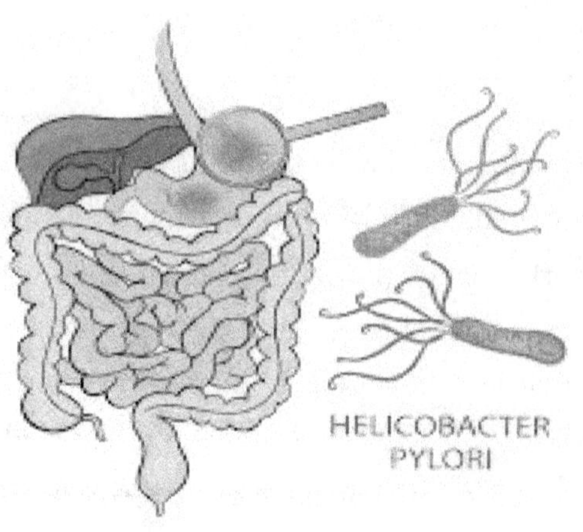

Numerous individuals have the microorganisms their whole lives and experience no manifestations. At the point when it causes incessant gastric aggravation and stays untreated, genuine intricacies may happen. These may incorporate draining ulcers and stomach disease. H. pylori are the principle hazard factor for certain kinds of stomach malignancy.

As indicated by the 1998 information from the CDC, annihilation paces of H. pylori are 61 to 94 percent; when a FDA-affirmed anti-microbial treatment is utilized. Rates are most elevated when anti-toxins are joined with a corrosive reducer. Including regular medicines may offer extra recuperating benefits.

What you can do now?

In the United States, specialists only sometimes test for H. pylori except if you have side effects. In the event that you have indications, call your primary care physician for an assessment. H. pylori contamination imparts indications to other stomach conditions, for example, indigestion and

GERD. It's significant you get the correct conclusion to ensure you're dealt with accurately.

If you test positive for H. pylori, the earlier you begin treatment, the more improvement you get. Normal medicines aren't probably going to hurt you, yet they aren't demonstrated to kill the disease. Try not to utilize them rather than regular medicines without your PCP's management.

Step by step instructions to forestall future contamination

The wellspring of H. pylori is muddled. There are no proper proposals from the CDC to forestall it. When all is said in done, you should rehearse great cleanliness by habitually washing your hands and appropriately setting up your food. In case you're in the likelihood of having H. pylori, complete your full course of treatment to decrease your danger of repeat.

CHAPTER FIVE

H. PYLORI PLUS PEPTIC ULCER AS WELL AS HOW IT BRINGS ABOUT PEPTIC ULCER, AND THE SYMPTOMS

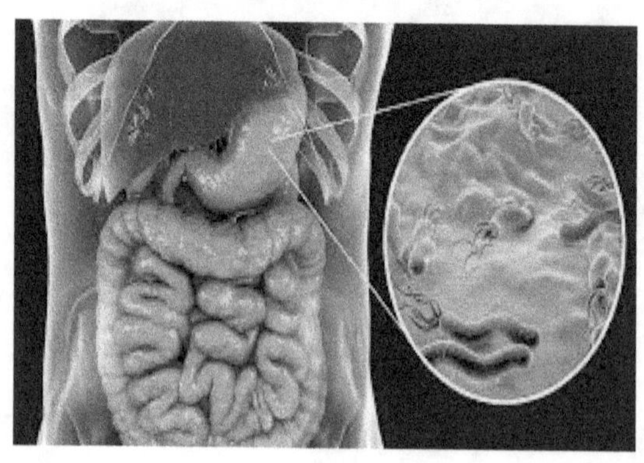

Meaning of a peptic ulcer

A peptic ulcer is a sore on the covering of the stomach or duodenum, which is the start of the small digestive system. Peptic ulcers are normal: One out of 10 Americans builds up an ulcer sooner or later in their life. One reason for peptic ulcer is bacterial contamination; however a few ulcers are brought about by long haul utilization of non-steroidal mitigating specialists (NSAIDs), like anti-inflamatory medicine and ibuprofen. In a couple of cases, dangerous tumors in the stomach or pancreas can cause ulcers. Peptic ulcers are not brought about by pressure or eating fiery food.

As was explained earlier on Helicobacter pylorus (H. pylori) is a sort of microbes. Specialists accept that H. pylori is answerable for most of peptic ulcers, just as constant gastritis (irritation of the stomach lining) and conceivably gastric disease.

H. pylori disease is normal in the United States: About 20 percent of individuals fewer than 40 years of age and half of those more than 60 years have it. Most contaminated individuals, nonetheless, don't create ulcers. Why H. pylori don't cause ulcers in each tainted individual isn't known. In all probability, disease relies upon attributes of the contaminated individual, the sort of H. pylori, and different factors yet to be found.

Scientists are not sure how individuals contract H. pylori, yet they figure it might be through food or water.

Specialists have discovered H. pylori in the spit of some tainted individuals, so the microscopic organisms may likewise spread through mouth-to-mouth contact, for example, kissing.

How do H. pylori cause a peptic ulcer?

The H. pylori microorganism debilitates the defensive mucous covering of the stomach and duodenum, in this manner permitting corrosive to break through to the touchy coating underneath. Both the corrosive and the microbes disturb the covering and cause a sore, or ulcer.

H. pylori can make due in stomach corrosive since it secretes proteins that kill the corrosive. This component permits H. pylori to advance toward the "sheltered" region – the defensive mucous coating. Once there, the bacterium's winding shape causes it tunnel through the coating.

What are the indications of an ulcer?

Stomach distress is the most widely recognized indication. This distress generally:

-is a dull, chewing throb.

-travels every way for a few days or weeks.

-happens 2 to 3 hours after a feast.

-happens in the night (when the stomach is unfilled).

-is soothed by eating.

-is soothed by acid neutralizer prescriptions.

Different manifestations incorporate

-weight reduction

-helpless craving

-swelling

-burping

-queasiness

-retching

A few people experience truth be told, mellow indications or none by any means.

Crisis Symptoms

On the off chance that you have any of these indications, summon your primary care physician right:

Sharp, unexpected, tenacious stomach torment.

Wicked or dark stools.

Wicked regurgitation or regurgitation that appears as though espresso beans.

They could be indications of a difficult issue, for example,

Hole – when the ulcer tunnels through the stomach or duodenal divider.

Dying – when corrosive or the ulcer breaks a vein.

Deterrent – when the ulcer hinders the way of food attempting to leave the stomach.

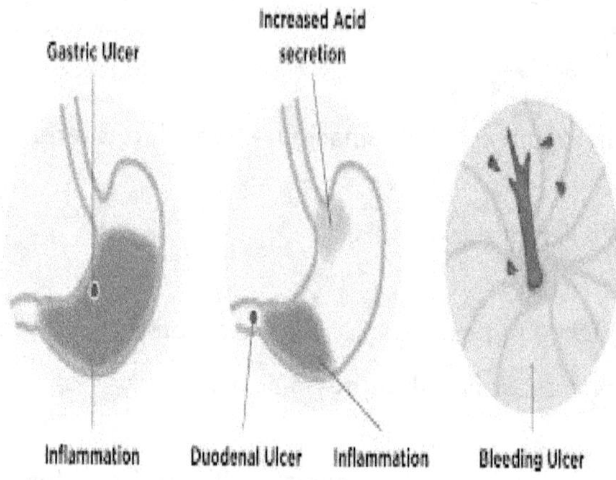

CHAPTER SIX

HOW IS A H. PYLORI-RELATED ULCER ANALYZED, OTHER DIAGNOSIS, TREATMENTS OF H. PYLORI PEPTIC ULCERS AND OTHER FACTS?

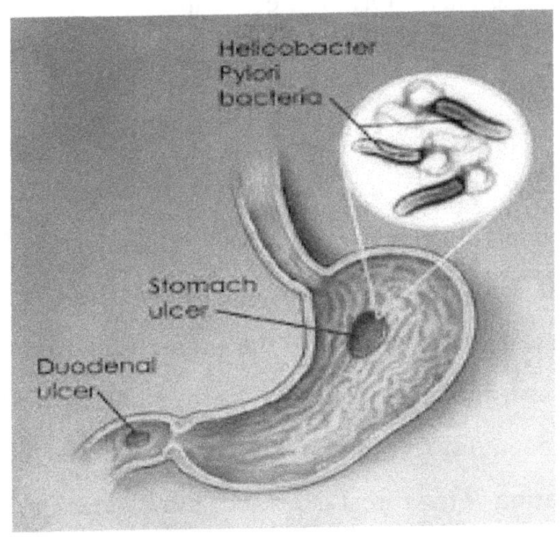

Diagnosing a Ulcer

To see whether indications are brought about by a ulcer, the specialist may do an upper gastrointestinal (GI) arrangement or an endoscopy.

Upper GI arrangement — An x-beam of the throat, stomach, and duodenum. The patient beverages a powdery fluid, called barium, to make these organs and any ulcers appear all the more unmistakably on the x-beam.

Endoscopy — A test that utilizes an endoscope, a slender, lit cylinder with a small camera on the end. The patient is gently quieted, and the specialist cautiously slips the endoscope into the mouth and down the throat to the stomach and duodenum. This permits the specialist to see the coating of the throat, stomach, and duodenum. The specialist can utilize the endoscope to take photographs of ulcers or eliminate a little bit of tissue to see under a magnifying lens.

Diagnosing H. pylori You Should Know

In the event that a ulcer is discovered, the specialist will test the patient for H. pylori. This test is significant in light of the fact that treatment for a ulcer brought about by H. pylori is not the same as that for a ulcer brought about by NSAIDs.

H. pylori are analyzed through blood, breath, stool, and tissue tests. Blood tests are generally normal. They recognize antibodies to H. pylori microorganisms. Blood is taken at the specialist's office through a finger stick.

Urea breath tests are a compelling indicative strategy for H. pylori. They are likewise utilized after treatment to see whether it worked. In the specialist's office, the patient beverages a urea arrangement that contains an uncommon carbon molecule. On the off chance that H. pylori are available, it separates the urea, delivering the carbon. The blood conveys the carbon to the lungs, where the patient breathes out it. The breath test is 96 percent to 98 percent precise.

Stool tests might be utilized to identify H. pylori contamination in the patient's faecal issue. Studies have demonstrated that this test, called the Helicobacter pylori stool antigen (HpSA) test, is exact for diagnosing H. pylori.

Tissue tests are typically done utilizing the biopsy test that is taken out with the endoscope. There are three sorts:

The fast urease test identifies the protein urease, which is created by H. pylori.

A histology test (or biopsy) permits the specialist to discover and look at the real microbes.

A culture test includes permitting H. pylori to develop in the tissue test.

In diagnosing H. pylori, blood, breath, and stool tests are regularly done before tissue tests since they are less intrusive. Be that as it may, blood tests are not used to distinguish H. pylori following treatment in light of the fact that a patient's blood can show positive outcomes even after H. pylori has been wiped out.

How are H. pylori peptic ulcers treated?

Medications Used to Treat H. pylori Peptic Ulcers

Anti-infection agents: metronidazole, antibiotic medication, clarithromycin, amoxicillin

H2 blockers: cimetidine, ranitidine, famotidine, nizatidine

Proton siphon inhibitors: omeprazole, lansoprazole, rabeprazole, esomeprazole, pantoprozole

Stomach-lining defender: bismuth subsalicylate

H. pylori peptic ulcers are treated with drugs that slaughter the microbes, decrease stomach corrosive, and ensure the stomach lining. Anti-toxins are utilized to execute the microorganisms. Two sorts of corrosive smothering medications may be utilized: H2 blockers and proton siphon inhibitors.

H2 blockers work by blocking histamine, which invigorates corrosive emission. They help decrease ulcer torment following half a month. Proton siphon inhibitors smother corrosive creation by ending the system that siphons the corrosive into the stomach. H2 blockers and proton siphon inhibitors have been endorsed alone for a considerable length of time as medicines for ulcers. Yet, utilized alone, these medications don't annihilate H. pylori and in this manner don't fix H. pylori - related ulcers. Bismuth subsalicylate, a segment of Pepto-Bismol, is utilized to shield the stomach lining from corrosive. It additionally slaughters H. pylori.

Treatment as a rule includes a blend of anti-microbial, corrosive silencers, and stomach defenders. Anti-toxin regimens suggested for patients may contrast across locales of the world on the grounds that various zones have started to show protection from specific anti-toxins.

The utilization of just a single medicine to treat H. pylori isn't suggested. As of now, the most demonstrated powerful treatment is a 2-week course of treatment called triple treatment. It includes taking two anti-toxins to execute the microorganisms and either a corrosive silencer or stomach-lining shield. Fourteen day triple treatment diminishes ulcer manifestations, kills the microscopic organisms, and forestalls ulcer repeat in excess of 90 percent of patients.

Sadly, patients may discover triple treatment confused on the grounds that it includes taking upwards of 20 pills per day. Likewise, the anti-infection agents utilized in triple treatment may cause mellow reactions, for example, queasiness, regurgitating, looseness of the bowels, dull stools, metallic intuition regarding the mouth, tipsiness, migraine, and yeast contamination in ladies. Most symptoms can be treated with prescription withdrawal. Nevertheless, late investigations show that fourteen days of triple treatment is ideal.

Early consequences of studies in different nations recommend that multi week of triple treatment might be as compelling as the 2-week treatment, with fewer reactions.

Another alternative is fourteen days of double treatment. Double treatment includes two medications: an anti-infection and a corrosive silencer. It isn't as viable as triple treatment.

Fourteen days of fourfold treatment, which utilizes two anti-microbial, a corrosive silencer, and a stomach-lining shield, glances promising in research consider. It is additionally called bismuth triple treatment.

Can H. pylori disease be forestalled?

Nobody knows without a doubt how H. pylori spread, so counteraction is troublesome. Analysts are attempting to build up an immunization to forestall contamination.

For what reasons don't all specialists consequently check for H. pylori?

Changing clinical convictions and practice requires some serious energy. For almost 100 years, researchers and specialists believed that ulcers were brought about by pressure, hot food, and liquor. Treatment included bed rest and a tasteless eating routine. Afterward, analysts added stomach corrosive to the rundown of causes and started treating ulcers with acid neutralizers.

Since H. pylori was found in 1982, considers led far and wide have indicated that utilizing anti-toxins to pulverize H. pylori fixes peptic ulcers. The pervasiveness of H. pylori ulcers is evolving. The contamination is getting more uncommon in individuals conceived in created nations. The clinical network, be that as it may, keeps on discussing H. pylori function in peptic ulcers. In the event that you have a peptic ulcer and have not been tried for H. pylori disease, converse or relate with your primary care physician.

Things to Remember

A peptic ulcer is a sore in the covering of the stomach or duodenum.

Most of peptic ulcers are brought about by the H. pylori bacterium. A considerable lot of different cases are brought about by NSAIDs (a class of agony reliever). None are brought about by fiery food or stress.

H. pylori can be sent from individual to individual through close contact and introduction to upchuck.

Continuously wash your hands in the wake of utilizing the restroom and before eating.

A mix of anti-microbials and different medications is the best treatment for H. pylori peptic ulcers

Your PCP may likewise perform numerous different tests and methods to help affirm their analysis:

Physical test

During a physical test, your PCP will look at your stomach to check for indications of swelling, delicacy, or agony. They'll additionally tune in for any sounds inside the mid-region.

Blood test

You may need to give blood tests, which will be utilized to search for antibodies against H. pylori. For a blood test, a medical services supplier will draw a limited quantity of blood from your arm or hand. The blood will at that point be sent to a research facility for examination. This is just useful in the event that you have never been treated for H. pylori previously.

Stool test

A faeces test might be expected to check for indications of H. pylori in your excrement. Your primary care physician will give you a compartment to bring home with you to catch and store an example of your stool. When you return the compartment to your medical services supplier, they will send the example to a research centre for examination. This and the breath tests typically will expect you to stop prescriptions, for example, anti-microbial and proton siphon inhibitors (PPIs) before the test.

Breath test

In the event that you have a breath test, you'll swallow an arrangement containing urea. On the off chance that H. pylori microbes are available, they will deliver a catalyst that separates this blend and will deliver carbon dioxide, which a unique gadget at that point recognizes.

Endoscopy

On the off chance that you have an endoscopy, your primary care physician will embed a long, slender instrument called an endoscope into your mouth and down into your stomach and duodenum. A joined camera will send back pictures on a screen for your primary care physician to see. Any irregular regions will be assessed. In the event that essential, exceptional apparatuses utilized with the endoscope will permit your PCP to take tests from these territories.

What are the confusions of H. pylori diseases?

H. pylori contaminations can prompt peptic ulcers, however the disease or the ulcer itself can prompt more genuine complexities. These include:

Inner dying, which can happen when a peptic ulcer gets through your vein and is related with iron inadequacy weakness deterrent, which can happen when something like a tumour hinders the food from leaving your stomach

Hole, which can happen when a ulcer gets through your stomach divider peritonitis, which is a contamination of the peritoneum, or the covering of the stomach pit

Modern research shows that tainted individuals likewise have an expanded danger of stomach disease. While the contamination is a significant reason for stomach malignant growth, the vast majority tainted with H. pylori never create stomach disease.

How are H. pylori diseases treated?

On the off chance that you have a H. pylori contamination that isn't causing you any issues and you aren't at expanded danger of stomach disease, treatment may not offer any advantages.

Stomach malignancy, alongside duodenal and stomach ulcers, is related with H. pylori disease. On the off chance that you have close family members with stomach disease or an issue, for example, a stomach or duodenal ulcer, your PCP may need you to have treatment. Therapy can fix a ulcer, and it might diminish your danger of creating stomach malignancy.

CHAPTER SEVEN

WAY OF LIFE AND DIET, AND OTHER FACTS YOU NEED TO KNOW, AND CONCLUSION

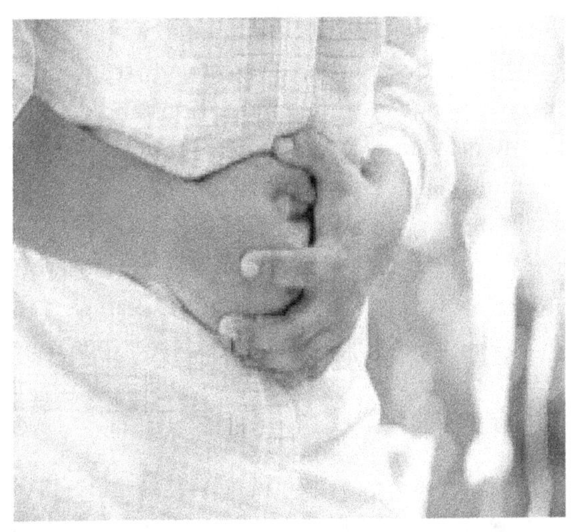

There's no proof that food and nourishment assume a part in forestalling or causing peptic ulcer sickness in individuals contaminated with H. pylori. Notwithstanding, hot nourishments, liquor, and smoking may decline a peptic ulcer and keep it from recuperating appropriately.

What would I be able to expect in the long haul?

For some, individuals contaminated with H. pylori, their diseases never create any troubles. In case you're encountering indications and get treatment, your drawn out viewpoint is commonly sure. At any rate a month in the wake of completing your treatment, your PCP will check to ensure it worked. Contingent upon your age and other clinical issues, your PCP may utilize a urea or stool test to check whether your treatment worked.

On the off chance that you create illnesses related with a H. pylori contamination, your standpoint will rely upon the ailment, how soon it's analyzed, and how it's dealt with. You may

need to take more than one round of treatment
to execute the H. pylori microbes.

On the off chance that the disease is as yet
present after one round of therapy, a peptic ulcer
could return or, all the more infrequently,
stomach malignancy could create. Not many
individuals contaminated with H. pylori will
create stomach malignancy. In any case, on the
off chance that you have a family background of
stomach malignancy, you ought to get testing
and treatment for H. pylori disease.

Conclusion

Lastly, the rules to getting the expected results as
regards Helicobacter Pylori cure are the right
applications as well as the guidelines explained in
this breath-taking guide. Therefore, the
guidelines and instructions should be strictly
followed to get the optimum and curative results.
And always consult your doctor when the need
arises.

Good luck to you as you commence!

THE END